Wellness

Body, Mind and Soul

Wellness

Body, Mind and Soul

Geetha Patel

SUNSTONE PRESS

SANTA FE

Sunstone books may be purchased for educational, business, or sales promotional use. For information please write: Special Markets Department, Sunstone Press, P.O. Box 2321, Santa Fe, New Mexico 87504-2321.

Book and cover design › Vicki Ahl
Body typeface › Adobe Caslon Pro
Printed on acid-free paper
∞
eBook 978-1-61139-439-9

Library of Congress Cataloging-in-Publication Data

Names: Patel, Geetha, 1944- author.
Title: Wellness : body, mind and soul / by Geetha Patel.
Description: Santa Fe : Sunstone Press, [2015]
Identifiers: LCCN 2015041481 | ISBN 9781632930989 (softcover : alk. paper)
Subjects: LCSH: Health--Popular works. | Nutrition. | Vitality. | Self-care,
  Health.
Classification: LCC RA776 .P25 2015 | DDC 613.2--dc23
LC record available at http://lccn.loc.gov/2015041481

SUNSTONE PRESS IS COMMITTED TO MINIMIZING OUR ENVIRONMENTAL IMPACT ON THE PLANET. THE PAPER USED IN THIS BOOK IS FROM RESPONSIBLY MANAGED FORESTS. OUR PRINTER HAS RECEIVED CHAIN OF CUSTODY (COC) CERTIFICATION FROM: THE FOREST STEWARDSHIP COUNCIL™ (FSC®), PROGRAMME FOR THE ENDORSEMENT OF FOREST CERTIFICATION™ (PEFC™), AND THE SUSTAINABLE FORESTRY INITIATIVE® (SFI®). THE FSC® COUNCIL IS A NON-PROFIT ORGANIZATION, PROMOTING THE ENVIRONMENTALLY APPROPRIATE, SOCIALLY BENEFICIAL AND ECONOMICALLY VIABLE MANAGEMENT OF THE WORLD'S FORESTS. FSC® CERTIFICATION IS RECOGNIZED INTERNATIONALLY AS A RIGOROUS ENVIRONMENTAL AND SOCIAL STANDARD FOR RESPONSIBLE FOREST MANAGEMENT.

WWW.SUNSTONEPRESS.COM
SUNSTONE PRESS / POST OFFICE BOX 2321 / SANTA FE, NM 87504-2321 /USA
(505) 988-4418 / ORDERS ONLY (800) 243-5644 / FAX (505) 988-1025

I would like to dedicate this book to
my wonderful late mother, Cecilia and
the elders in my community back in Soouth India who
helped me put together this book.

Contents

Foreword

"Health is a state of complete physical, mental and social well being, and not merely the absence of disease or infirmity."
—World Health Organization 1948

I was in my early forties when I immigrated to Canada with my family. The buzz about health foods and eating healthy was making its way into mainstream Canadians. Even though people were watching their diets and trying to lose weight, there was not a conscious search for the secrets to good health and happiness. As the World Health Organization rightly points out, health is a total package of well being of body, mind, and soul. Whenever the topic of eating healthy, longevity and happiness came up, I could not but think of my neighbour back in India. Let me call her Genevieve aunty. She was past seventy and was not only in excellent health, active, and on no medications, but also looked amazingly young for her age and had a positive attitude toward life. It is not that she did not have her share of trials and tribulations, but the way she handled them, always looking at the brighter side, is what made her who she was. I had known her since I was a child. In India we address every lady our mother's age as 'aunty,' so we too called her aunty. She came to Canada to be with her children a few years after I arrived.

It was then that I realized that Genevieve aunty, and the other healthy and happy elders must be doing something right. I wanted to know their secret. This thought inspired me to talk to the elderly in Canada and India to see what they thought contributed toward their health and well being.

When I spoke to Genevieve aunty, she just laughed at me and said, "Perhaps it is because of the genes I inherited from my parents.

"Could very well be, I said, "but I would like to know your childhood and upbringing, your food and your lifestyle, your beliefs and your attitude that might have contributed to your state of health now."

She replied, "You are indeed asking me a lot, but I'll try and answer your question to the best of my recollection. Come over when you have time and I will tell you what I remember about my life. Please remember there are no guarantees in life about anything, including health. Many factors come into play in each person's life and there is no magic wand. I don't know what will happen tomorrow, but I am grateful to God for these seventy plus years. I will tell you about my life, my beliefs and attitude. It does not mean that it is the only way to well being, but it has been my way."

We talked a lot after that; sometimes for hours and I enjoyed every minute of it. The more I heard, the more I felt that these things were worth recording. She had a life that was in harmony with nature. The best part was, all the natural remedies she used for simple ailments, were also used by my mother, when I was growing up in India. After all she and my mother were almost of the same age and their parents had the same upbringing.

After that, I interviewed many other elderly healthy people and took notes. Very soon I noticed that there were about five to six factors that were common to most of them. I knew then that it couldn't be a coincidence.

Many of those I talked to or interviewed have passed away, including Genevieve aunty, my mother, Mrs. Shah and more, but I will never forget their advice and their zest for life.

Preface

Wellness: Body, Mind, and Soul is a book that touches on the common elements that contribute towards the well being of a person. Ancient wisdom dictates that all we need to keep ourselves healthy is found in nature, and that is what our ancestors did to maintain their health. Thomas Edison had the foresight and conviction when he said that "the doctors of the future will no longer treat the human frame with drugs, but rather will cure and prevent disease with nutrition."

Growing up in the natural surroundings of South India, Geetha Patel vividly recalls some of the most interesting anecdotes of ailments in her life and those of her loved ones, and how they were dealt with and treated in her household and community. Geetha Patel also shares the factors that have contributed towards her own health and well being, while educating the readers of the medicinal values of herbs that are easily and abundantly found in Canada. She encourages readers to value this precious life by having the right belief and attitude, living an active life, and eating healthy. The recipes at the end of the book will inspire the readers to cook and eat dishes that are easy to make and are beneficial for maintaining good health.

> "Health is a state of complete harmony of the body, mind and spirit. When one is free from physical disabilities and mental distractions, the gates of the soul open."
>
> —B.K.S. Iyengar

Acknowledgements

My special thanks go to all the elderly ladies and gentlemen I interviewed during the course of many years here in Canada and back in India, who so readily shared the secrets to their good health and well being, with me. I would also like to thank my mother Cecelia, Genevieve aunty, and all the elders in my community for sharing their valuable knowledge with me.

The book would not have been possible without the constant encouragement, support, and the interest shown by my friends and colleagues.

1

Five Crucial Factors

*A*ccording to most healthy elderly people I have talked with, there were five crucial factors that perhaps contributed to their total well being.

Faith/Spirituality/Philosophy

> "That deep emotional conviction of the presence of a superior reasoning power, which is revealed in the incomprehensible universe, forms my idea of God."
>
> —Albert Einstein

Genevieve aunty was a Catholic and believed in God according to her religious beliefs, which was a path of love, forgiveness, justice, compassion, and equality as shown by Jesus Christ. It was a very important part of her life. However, every one I interviewed or talked to was not a Christian. There were Hindus, Muslims and Zoroastrians, but most of them had this faith in the existence of God or superior spiritual being, through their different religions, spirituality or just a way of life. This faith, they said was what helped them cope with all the trials and tribulations life threw at them from time to time, without losing hope and getting desperate.

"If God brings me to it, He will bring me through it."

Contentment and Gratitude

> "He who is not contented with what he has, would not be contented with what he would like to have."
>
> —Socrates

Most of them were also content with what they had and were grateful for the many blessings they enjoyed. Some said that constant craving for things one does not have and the desire and race to acquire them would cause undue stress both to the body and mind. Ambition is good only as long as it does not rob us of our peace of mind and sleep.

Forgiveness

"To forgive is the highest, most beautiful form of love. In return, you will receive untold peace and happiness."

—Robert Muller

They were of the opinion that having a clean and burden free heart which has forgiven all and has asked forgiveness from those offended or hurt by us intentionally or unintentionally, was very essential for good health. They believed that when a person harbours grudge, hate or anger towards another, it is he or she who suffers and not the one hated.

Healthy Lifestyle

"Let thy food be thy medicine and thy medicine be thy food."

—Hippocrates (460–377 B.C.)

Most of the people enjoyed cooking and eating. Since most of those I interviewed were born in the early twenties, they were fortunate enough to eat food that was unpolluted and home grown, especially in India. Since their pallets were used to home cooked meals, they continued to do so, paying more attention to a wholesome diet, no matter where they landed in their old age. They were also quite active, perhaps not in the sense of going to the gym and long walks, but doing constant housework, gardening and travelling everywhere by foot as that is what most of those born during those years, normally did. Then again there were a handful who ate what they wanted and yet were healthy. These perhaps were compensated with good genes, positive outlook on life and active lifestyle, or perhaps their bodies were simply able to absorb and digest food, better.

A Purpose in Life

> "The mystery of human existence lies not in just staying alive, but in finding something to live for."
>
> —Fyodor Dostoyevsky, *The Brothers Karamazov*

Every one of the elders I talked with had a purpose or focus in life. It didn't matter what the focus was. If one had discovered painting, the other was a writer; a third one had discovered love and so on. Each was happy to be alive and able to get up every morning. One elderly person said that her goal was to get her master's degree within three years and she was so enthusiastic about it that it would put any young person to shame. Some were even working on their childhood hobbies, but all of them had a purpose, and the zest to live.

> "If you can't figure out your purpose, figure out your passion. For your passion will lead you right into your purpose."
>
> —Bishop T.D. Jakes

About a quarter of them had a drink every day and were sexually active.

Genevieve aunty explained to me how these factors that I had discovered had played their role in her own personal life, too.

"Prayer and giving thanks were instilled in us. We believed that God was Omnipotent, Omniscient and Omnipresent. We also believed that God was all merciful, bountiful and powerful. We started our day by offering the day to God and ended it by giving thanks and asking for forgiveness for the errors committed during the day, knowingly or unknowingly. We were reminded that bread earned with honesty and integrity was far better than riches gained in a dishonest way. That, our parents said, was the only way to peace of mind, a good night's sleep and good health. Our parents told us to compare ourselves to people who had less than us, in order to realize our blessings. That did not mean that we had to passively accept the state we were in, but strive for the better with the means at our disposal without grudge or envy. My mother loved being a mother. Her life revolved around her family and she enjoyed it. My father loved and enjoyed his job. It was never a job for him; it was his purpose, his reason for living. I loved my job as a teacher. Now that I am retired, I love to paint. Above all, we used natural remedies for simple ailments."

I could not believe my ears. My mother brought us up exactly with the same beliefs and values. Like her, we too always resorted to natural remedies for ailments such as; stomach upset, minor sprains, constipation, diarrhea, headache, allergic rashes and so on. The food she ate growing up had a very important role to play in her good health. My life was no different. Everything we ate, as I was growing up, was natural and organic because it was home grown with just cow dung as manure.

When I was growing up, our food consisted of home grown fruits and vegetables, homebred chickens and their eggs. I remember feeding the chickens with grains every morning.
Our milk came from our field grazed cattle and butter, yogurt, buttermilk and ghee were made from this milk.

Fish was caught from the unpolluted streams or rivers. Honey was collected directly from the beehives in the trees. Honey or home-made jam was eaten with rice pancakes and crepes. Bananas were sliced and dried in the sun and preserved in honey and eaten as dessert after food. Vinegar and salt was our salad dressing. The fresh grated coconut that was used in our cooking came from our trees. The extra coconuts were dried to make oil. Some of the coconut powder that was left after extracting the oil was mixed with the cooked grains and overripe excess fruits and fed to the cattle. The rest was used as manure for the plants.

Once a year all of us had to drink some bitter liquid made from herbs to clean our stomachs. There were none of the preservatives in our food nor was any spray being used on the vegetables or fruits we grew and ate. It was sad that by the time I was a teenager, bug sprays were slowly being introduced to increase production. Hence my younger siblings became the victims of this pollution.

Then Genevieve aunty talked about her mother's role in ensuring that they ate the right food. Her mother was not literate, but had a wealth of knowledge about the right foods for the right time and age of a child or an adult. On the other hand, my mother was much more modern and literate. She was educated by the British and loved reading.

Here's what I remembered about my mother's role in ensuring that we her children remained healthy. 'Behind every healthy child is a healthy mother.' This saying is very true as far as my mother was concerned. Being a stay-home-mom, she devoted her life to her husband and children. She saw to it that we were fed nutritious food, were clean and had order and discipline in our lives. There weren't the present day temptations from TV ads enticing children to eat food that may not be good for them nor there were busy working mothers trying to cope with the pressures of work and home that many a times is the reason for eating fast food for dinner. Times surely have changed and it is very challenging though not impossible to organize home cooked meals every day.

Our lunch from Monday to Saturday usually consisted of unpolished brown rice, fish curry, vegetables and salad. Fresh coconut was used both in the curry and vegetable and coconut oil was used in cooking. The coconuts came from our trees and the oil was extracted from our coconuts. Hence it was all organic. Sunday was meat day, when we had chicken, lamb or pork instead of fish. Our mother was a voracious reader and as a result, we her children had to eat whatever the books said was good for health. As we were growing up, our mother gave us sprouted raw lotus seeds, every morning. They did not taste the greatest, but she said that they were full of vitamin B Complex and hence good for us. We had no say in this. We had to just follow orders. Then it became raw tomato every morning before breakfast. Now I sprout the seeds and use them in salads, soups or just stir fry them with onions, garlic, tomatoes, walnuts and green chillies and eat them semi raw. I sometimes add pieces of mango to this semi raw salad. You can sprout any kind of lentils as long as they are not split. (The recipe below explains how to sprout lentils.) Then, my mother discovered a new and unique porridge which was drunk in our house. This was the porridge she and my aunt drank until they died.

Genevieve aunty's mother unlike mine did not lay much emphasis on education. Since girls were to be married at an early age, only boys were encouraged to study. My mother however, loved knowledge and education. As a result, two of her girls became teachers, one bank manager and one a doctor. Education also played a very important part in our lives. She equated education to knowledge and knowledge to light. Without education, she said, our minds and souls will be clothed in the darkness of ignorance. "Prejudice is the child of ignorance," and that is why most of those who are prejudiced lack education. Therefore she kept herself abreast by reading whatever was available to her.

Both our mothers encouraged us to be outdoors when we could. 'A healthy mind in a healthy body,' she said. Hiking, playing "Seven Tiles" and catching crabs were some of the main fun activities we were involved in, during our vacations. We called hiking as "climbing the mountain." This hiking at an early age was good for our health and for building stamina. We started this hike as early as age nine or ten. We were not allowed to be outdoors from 12:30 to 4:00 pm, as she said that the sun was too strong at that time and that would be bad for the liver, as the sun produced too much bile. I don't know where she got this from, but we obeyed. When my father got back from work at noon, he was always given a glass of water with freshly squeezed lemon or butter milk to calm the bile, my mother said.

As cars were not in the picture during the time of my mother and even my time, we went to most of the places walking. During my time, cars were the luxuries of the few rich. We went walking to school, church and the doctor. During the holidays we went exploring nature and finding new streams, fruit trees, and even rocks with games carved on them. This was the most adventurous activity, of all. Our holidays were filled with physical activities, which kept us fit, healthy and happy. We learnt to adapt and innovate to occupy ourselves and enjoy ourselves. As far as I remember, there were very few obese people at that time.

We were out in the open as much as we could. I still remember climbing an eight foot square rock and seeing a game that we played with shells being carved on the top. We wondered how long ago this must have been carved and imagined children or perhaps adults sitting and playing this game. Those were good times. We were one with nature and our joys were simple and pure. We knew all the insects that flew or crawled. We were familiar with the different birds and their sounds. Woodpeckers, minas, parrots, owls, koels, sparrows, crows and bats were the common birds. We ate the wild berries when we found them and drank the clear spring water. If the berry tree was too high one of the brave boys would climb the tree and cut a branch and all of us would sit around this branch and eat the berries. These were the joys we once had, and are alien to my children and grandchildren.

Most of today's children have become couch potatoes playing video games or just watching the television or "the idiot box," as some old folks refer to it. It is essential therefore to enrol kids into sports or other activities such as dance and swimming so that they get enough physical exercise. So much has happened to ruin our health in just one generation around this world. Some may call those days backward, I call them divine. We lived how man was meant to live by his creator. Furthermore, working mothers neither have the time nor the energy required to provide the family with healthy home-cooked meals, unless they are organized and get the needed help from their husbands and growing children. As a result, many families are forced to resort to fast food dinners. However, when the family together makes healthy eating a priority and all hands contribute to make the work light, almost anything can be accomplished.

Neither my mother's generation nor I had any toys, except the ones made by carpenters. The board games in my time were; Snakes and Ladders, Chess, Ludo and Monopoly. We were allowed to play cards only during summer holidays, as cards were supposed to dull the mind compared to chess, which increased critical thinking and problem solving abilities. Usually, we played the board games either when it was raining or when it was too hot to go outside to play. The rest of the time, we were outside playing games that required a lot of physical activity.

Lunch was our main meal of the day, and we were all expected to rest for an hour or two after lunch, during holidays. Super was light, as we ate at about 8:00 pm and no activity was possible after that, as nine was bedtime. Now that I live in a commercial world, where it is very difficult or practically impossible to eat and drink the pure stuff I once did, I do what I can to remain healthy with the means I have.

It has been almost twenty years since I first started this project. Genevieve aunty, my mother and many I interviewed have passed away. I am now seventy and by the grace of God, am healthy, active, with no ailments and no medication. Therefore I have decided to write this book not only to share what I have been able to find out about the factors that might have contributed towards my good health and well being and that of many others, but also share other useful information that I have collected or recall from my childhood, that could be beneficial for others. For the most part in my life, I have eaten home cooked meals and have tried to cook everything from scratch. It is not only healthier but also much cheaper to cook your own meals. The following chapters will have natural remedies that we used for some simple ailments, growing up in India, foods and spices with medicinal values, homemade beauty treatments and even some healthy recipes, vegetarian and non- vegetarian. Since we live in a multicultural society, I have included recipes from many different nationalities. I have modified most of them to suit my taste. Many of them are improvised depending on what was in my fridge at that moment. That is what I want you to do. You can always substitute ingredients or even omit them altogether once you gain enough confidence.

Life however, while being the greatest gift, does not come with any guarantees. Even after eating healthy and being active one can fall ill. That is because other factors like our genes, hereditary factors and the environment we live in, play their part. We live only once in this world and therefore it is very important to satisfy our taste buds once in a while even if it means we are eating unhealthy food. Constant deprivation of something will make us crave for it more and more. It is therefore better to indulge ourselves time to time, in moderation, so that we don't go crazy with want of them. A piece of advice is; try not to go grocery shopping when hungry or eat sweets and desserts before a meal.

"There are those people who can eat one piece of chocolate, one piece of cake, drink one glass of wine. There are even people who smoke one or two cigarettes a week. And then there are people for whom one of anything is not even an option."

—Abigail Thomas, *Thinking About Memoir*

We should live every minute of this gift of life and not just exist. That is what most of the elderly I interviewed did and so do I. Genevieve aunty never lost her interest in learning new recipes or a new technique in painting. I also take every opportunity to enjoy life to the fullest. Like many elderly who had a purpose in their lives, I have found mine in writing.

Mrs. Shah, a senior lady from India once said to me, "My experience in life has taught me that as long as we live, we will feel. The feeling doesn't always have to be positive and uplifting. It can be sad and hurtful, yet it is something that we feel. The minute we stop feeling we are dead in our souls and spirits, even though our bodies may be alive. I learnt not to worry about the future or regret about the past, as neither are in my power to change. I have learnt to live today to the fullest because that is all we really have. As long as my happiness falls within the framework of righteousness, I don't think twice about having fun and enjoying myself."

What wise advice, I thought. Her speech reminded me of the quotation, "Forget yesterday—it has already forgotten you. Don't worry about the tomorrow you haven't even met. Instead, open your eyes and your heart to a truly precious gift: today." (Steve Maraboli, *Life, the Truth, and Being Free)*

Mrs. Hollands from Canada was another true inspiration to me. Her positive attitude and her constant remark, "I had a good life; I loved a lot and was loved by many," made me always admire her. She too had some advice for me about health: "Health should not be our obsession, but just the result of a way of our life. Weight should not be equated with good health. One can be really healthy with a little under or over weight, as long as one is not too fat or thin. The minute health and weight become an obsession, we fail to live fully."

How true her words were! She said that she always ate a well balanced diet and enjoyed the food she cooked. She also loved baking and enjoyed eating those goodies she baked. Once again I was reminded of Lewis Thomas'

(*The Medusa and the Snail*) words: "As a people, we have become obsessed with Health. There is something fundamentally, radically unhealthy about all this. We do not seem to be seeking more exuberance in living as much as staving off failure, putting off dying. We have lost all confidence in the human body."

2

Remedies for Unique Conditions

*I*n this chapter I will tell you about the simple remedies we used in my household and my community in India. Some of them are unique. I have already told you that I am in excellent health. I weigh about 143 pounds and am 5'5" tall, which may not be the ideal height and weight as per the present day beauty standard requirements, but am quite happy with it. I also share the five factors which most of the seniors I interviewed, pointed out as being the keys to their well being.

I cannot categorically say that the remedies were all successful at all times. There were times when these remedies did not work and we needed intervention from the doctors, and we got that intervention. However, most of the time these remedies worked for common cold, fever, stomach pain, sinus, sprains and allergies.

I still remember my mother grinding small brown Ayurvedic pills in water and a drop of liquor and putting it on the tongue of my siblings when they were just a few days old. I still remember how healthy, plump and happy my siblings were. The babies never had any allopathic medicine, except the very important vaccinations such as small pox and polio, until the age of three or four. The only time there was a visit to the doctor was when there was something major like my sister getting rheumatic fever or when I got Malaria at the age of two. Every one of us had measles, mumps and chicken pox by the time we were eight or nine. No medicine was given for this. When the fever went too high, my mother put cold compresses on our forehead. We were given only rice congee and pickle until we were completely alright. She nursed us tenderly and waited patiently for our sickness to run its course, attending to us with great love and care. Only after complete recovery, we were given a bath and normal food to eat. Besides simple ailments there were remedies even for some unique conditions.

Getting Rid of Fright in Children: True Story

Some children get very scared when they hear any loud noise. They literally jump up in their seats or in their beds. I was one of those children who was very scared of the slightest noise. I am sure there was a psychological reason for this, which of course, no one was aware. You may be surprised to know that there was a remedy for that too. There were times when all of us children and women sat around the grinding stone. This grinding stone was made up of two circular polished heavy stones placed one on the top of the other (similar to the one seen at the Pioneer Village). The top stone had a wooden handle inserted tightly on the top and a hole in the centre. Grain, especially, roasted rice of about two tablespoons would be poured into this hole, at one time. One person (usually a woman) would then turn the top stone slowly, so that the rice could be ground. The flour would then pour out, from between the two stones. A clean white cloth would be placed below the stones to collect the flour. This flour was then used to make Christmas sweets. That was our mill those days. This was a long and tedious process and the older women took turns turning the stone. The children were there to listen to the stories, which were being told to lighten the chore.

At that time, a servant would be instructed to heat an iron rod to crimson red and placed in a brass pot. It would then be slowly brought behind where I (or any child with the same problem) was sitting and coldwater would be poured on the rod. This would create so much noise that people would naturally be surprised. There would be a safe distance between the child and the pot. The first time they did it, I jumped up so high and gave such a blood curdling scream, that my father came running to see what had happened. The second time my screams were less and by the fourth time, I had hardly noticed the noise. This got rid of my fright for noises. Though this may sound primitive, it had cured my fright. I am sure it has a psychological explanation.

Cure for Stammering: True Story

When my son was four years old, he suddenly developed stammering.

It was bizarre that a boy who spoke fluently should all of a sudden start stammering. I was devastated. Later on, I found out that my brother-in-law, with whom we lived at that time and who loved my children dearly, was trying to shoo a lizard (which are found on the walls of Indian homes) with a long stick. At the time he was also carrying my son in one hand. I heard that the lizard fell down and my son was so scared that he screamed with fright and the stammering started after that.

After the initial shock, I sat and thought about what I should do. Of course the first thing I did was knelt down and prayed to God to cure my son. People said that I should go to Mount Mary's church in Bombay and offer a candle in the shape of a tongue. Yes. I did that too. I would do anything for my son. Besides I did have faith in Mother Mary. I had now covered my faith base. I knew I had to do more. I prayed again for guidance. A plan came to my mind. I went to the bookstore and bought some books with the pictures of lizards and snakes and started reading about them to my son. Initially he did not want to even look at the picture of a lizard. I did not force him. I continued this talk about the animals including the lizard every day for a few minutes. Gradually he not only looked at the picture but was also ready to touch the picture. Then I went one step further. I brought two plastic lizards. I called them 'mama lizard' and 'baby lizard.' I made up good stories about them. We talked daily and played the lizard game. Eventually, my son held the lizard in his hand. In the mean time his stammering had started becoming less and less. Then I told him that when his uncle tried to shoo the lizard with a stick, it must have hurt the poor creature and it must have lost balance and fallen down to the floor.

"Can you imagine how frightened the poor lizard must have been?" I asked "The poor baby lizard must have been frightened and sad too."

He was very sympathetic toward the poor lizard and he held the lizard in his hands and apologized to it. He even kissed the plastic lizard. All this did not happen in a day. It must have taken more than a month or two. By then, his stammering had stopped completely. I did go to 'Mount Mary's Church' once again to light a candle of thanks. I was not a psychologist. Therefore I think God alone must have given me the wisdom to use such a strategy to cure my son's stammering. I was thankful. By gradually getting rid of the very fear that caused stammering, my son was cured. I don't know if this method was practised by all, but that is what I did.

Dealing with Hurts and Pains of the Heart: True Story

Every human being in this world experiences hurt and it stays deep in our hearts. Some incidents in our lives trigger this hurt and we feel very sad and almost depressed. I was no exception to this. There were little things that caused me a lot of hurt when I was growing up. I would push them somewhere under the conscious mind as you cannot really cast them away. There were times when something would trigger to bring those hurts to the surface. This happened more during my teenage years. Hence, I devised a plan to cope with this. When the burden of pain became intolerable, I would assign that night to dig into my heart and bring all the incidents of hurt I experienced, to the surface. This would fill my heart with so much pain that I would cry until all the pain was gone from my heart. By the time I fell asleep, my pillow would be soaked in my tears. However, when I got up the next day I was as good as new for a long time, until some trigger brought about the sadness again, and I assigned another night for crying. Perhaps being in the boarding school from an early age, I had to learn to cope with many things and find ways of dealing with things on my own. Eventually I got stronger and was able to remember those incidents without feeling sad and hurt, but in an objective manner. I knew that some of the things people said and did to me were wrong, but it did not hurt me, any more. Don't get me wrong. There was no sexual abuse. The physical punishment though common those days, did not bother me either, as all of us got straps for a bad report card, complaint from the teacher or even for back answering our parents. It was the hurtful remarks made by my mother, friends and siblings that hurt me the most. People could call it psychological therapy. It worked for me and I am sure it would work for all as long as they are able to bear the pain that will seize their hearts when they reminiscent these hurtful incidents. Today, I deal with issues right away and do not push them back to the sub conscience.

3

Natural Foods with Significant Medicinal Values

"This large and expensive stock of drugs will be unnecessary. The common resources of the lancet, a garden, a kitchen, fresh air, cool water, exercise, will be sufficient to cure all the diseases that are at present under the power of medicine."

—Benjamin Rush, MD

Elders in my community, including my mother and Genevieve aunty were glad to tell me the medicinal values of the natural foods that are found in abundance and are affordable. She said that it is very beneficial to use natural herbs and spices rather than the ready mix powders in our cooking. They said that fresh ginger, garlic, green chillies and herbs are excellent for health.

Ginger is very good for all digestive problems and for nausea. Eating a small piece of ginger after every meal will enhance your digestive process. My mother would give us a piece of ginger with a pinch of salt whenever we suffered nausea. We always ate a piece of ginger whenever our stomachs were upset. Have a glass of water ready, if you are not used to eating raw ginger. Start with a very tiny piece.

Slice a 3" long piece of ginger and soak it in a glass bottle with four tablespoons of honey and leave it for an hour or two. The juice from the ginger will come out and get mixed with the honey. Have a teaspoon of this liquid when you have cold. You can eat the ginger as well and use this 'ginger honey' in your tea. Use fresh grated ginger in all your recipes, even homemade soups.

Boil Crushed piece of ginger (2" long) and 3 cups of water for 30 minutes, then squeeze a lemon and add honey. Drink this mixture hot, 1/4 cup at a time, three times a day for cough and cold (morning, noon and bedtime). It even opens up the nasal passage and lets you sleep well.

Children between 5 and 12 can have less than 1/4 cup at a time. If you are not used to ginger, boil the ginger for a shorter time.

Try applying a mixture of ginger powder and hot water over the eyebrows for sinus. This stops the throbbing pain. This was my sister-in-law's remedy for her sinus. It may not work if the sinus is severe. Try very little, as it burns.

Garlic acts as a blood thinner and therefore good for controlling blood pressure. Eating raw garlic early in the morning to control blood pressure is practised throughout India. Drinking plenty of water, eating healthy and exercise also help control blood pressure. If none of this works, then you may have to take a prescribed medication. This is only for those who are not on blood thinners and blood pressure medications. Remember to tell your doctor if you are taking raw garlic every morning especially if you are going in for any surgery.

Here are some suggestions for minor sprains. I was a very clumsy girl growing up. I would constantly bang my open toe to the threshold and sprain it. It would swell and become very painful. My mother would crush 2 cloves of garlic, heat them in coconut oil and apply it warm on my toe and cover it with a light bandage. She did this two to three times a day. Within a couple of days my toe would be healed completely.

Garlic boiled in coconut oil may also be very effective for ingrown toe nails. With a dropper put a drop where the ingrown toe nail troubles. Use as hot as you can take. This works well when the toenail just starts growing in and when the problem is not severe. Do this often for good results.

I've also heard that cholesterol can be reduced by drinking the water that is poured on four slices of ginger and two cloves of crushed garlic. Remember to pour boiling water on garlic and ginger and leave it overnight. Drink the strained water first thing in the morning.

Green chillies are full of vitamin C. Use them instead of chilli powder or black pepper.

Pomegranate skin can be soaked in a glass of boiling water for about fifteen minutes and drunk for diarrhoea. (For one to three year olds, 1/4 teaspoon.) You can increase the amount as the child gets older (not more than about 3 tablespoons for age 15 and about 5 tablespoons for adults.

Yogurt, rice, banana, clear soups and teas were also our foods for diarrhoea

Constipation and Other Problems: True Story:

When my neighbour's son was very young, he had severe constipation problem. Once, the parents even had to take him to the hospital. The doctor examined him and asked his mother to get a fizzy orange drink and give it to him and wait for 20 minutes. Low and behold, he passed the motion without any problem. Ever since then, this is what I try first before buying anything from the counter.

Lots of vegetables with fibre, fruits, fish and soups are also good for constipation. Avoid meat and wheat when you have constipation.

Though milk has proven to be bad for cold and cough, it has a soothing effect when you drink hot milk with honey and a pinch of turmeric powder. Turmeric milk is famous throughout India. (Boil milk with a pinch of turmeric powder and then add honey. You can also add a piece of crushed ginger when boiling the milk). That is one of the cold medicines. Whenever we had severe cough and congestion in the chest, my mother would beat a raw egg, mix it with a glass of hot milk, honey and a spoon of brandy and give it to us for five consecutive mornings. It always worked.

Neem leaves are very bitter, but extremely good for cleansing your digestive system. Mahatma Gandhi used to eat Neem chutney (neem leaves ground with a little salt, chilly and tamarind), daily, with his meals.

Whenever children have measles, mumps or chicken pox, they are given small branches of Neem, to lightly brush on the skin to stop the itching and act as a disinfectant. Neem branches are even put in a vase in the room of the child, as it is supposed to purify the air. After measles and chicken Pox the children are bathed with water in which neem leaves are boiled. Boil a 1/2 or 1 cupful of neem leaves in a large pot filled with water. Then mix this water to a bucketful of warm water and pour this water on the body of the child as a final rinse and pat dry with a towel. This gets rid of all infection and any remaining itch.

Neem leaves are potent. You should never rub them directly on the skin. The skin can swell. Neem oil along with Cynth (an Ayurvedic oil)

is now being used in hospitals in India to prevent bedsores on bedridden patients.

True Story:

My very good friend's mother had a fall and broke her hip. She underwent surgery and was in intensive care for a fortnight due to complications. Though she recovered, she came home with a bad bedsore. All my friend was told to do was to dip cotton wool in neem oil and shove it inside the bedsore. The bedsore was completely healed within a month. Every day, the nurse sponged my friend's mother and applied neem oil to her whole body, and used an air mattress. She was bedridden for four more years and never got a bedsore again.

True Story:

My daughter was allergic to mosquito bites. She would swell up so badly that we had to rush her to the hospital, until I discovered the effects of Neem Oil on mosquito bites. After that, the minute she complained of a mosquito bite, I would apply a drop of neem oil and the bite would disappear within seconds and she never swelled up again as before. You can get it in the health food stores. It is very cheap in India.

Turmeric is another important spice used as remedy for many ailments. If we had a sore throat, we would add salt and a pinch of turmeric to warm water and gargle four or five times a day. Even the abscesses on gums were cured by mixing turmeric powder and salt and rubbing this mixture on the abscess for two to three days. My father never went to the dentist unless a natural remedy had not worked. He died at the age of seventy-seven and all his teeth were intact.

My father had told me that turmeric was antiseptic and it even helps stop bleeding.

True Story:

My father was a manager in a plantation. He told us that when he was young, he once accidentally slashed his ankle with a very sharp machete as he was trying to cut the branch of a coffee plant. Since the nearest doctor was many miles away and the only conveyance was the bullock cart, the people around him put turmeric on the wound, raised his foot and bandaged it and took him on that long journey to the hospital. It stopped the bleeding and his leg was saved. The doctor later said that it was the turmeric that stopped the infection, controlled the bleeding and helped in the healing process. Ever since I heard that story, turmeric has been used for every cut that my children or I have had.

Fenugreek seeds are known to have health values. Soaking a teaspoon full of these seeds overnight in 3/4 glass of water and drinking the water is not only good for health, but is also known to control diabetes. Don't ever substitute your medicine with this remedy when the sugar level is high, but do it along with your medication or when you just get a warning from your doctor.

One tablespoon of lightly toasted cumin seeds (Jira) can be eaten with a pinch of sugar when you lose your voice. Make three or four portions and eat at an interval of three to four hours. You'll be amazed how fast you get your voice back. Cumin seeds eaten with a pinch of salt are also useful in getting rid of gas and improving digestion.

In South India Jira Pani or Cumin Water is offered in restaurants during dinner. Here's how to prepare Jira Water. Boil 1tablespoon of Jira and asafoetida (Hing) powder each, in about one liter (34 ounces) of water for about 15 minutes and drink it with food. It is best to drink it warm. It is good for digestion. Make it fresh and drink it as often as you can or when your stomach is upset.

When you get cramps in your calves or toes, get up and walk. If they don't go away, drink one or two glasses of water. Dehydration causes cramps. Since I have been getting cramps since I was 14 years old, and have tried everything, and I have found that drinking water with a little sugar and a pinch of salt works for me.

Boil green chillies and garlic in equal proportion for at least an hour and spray the strained liquid on plants that have deceases or fungus. The chillies have to be really very pungent.

Ajwain and Sesame Seeds:

These seeds are tiny but have great medicinal value. Whenever there was minor stomach problem such as bloating, gas or indigestion, our mother gave us ajwain seeds to chew. These are quite hot in taste and may not be appropriate for those who are not used to it or children. Although chewing the seeds is the best way to eat them, you can also make ajwain tea by boiling 1 tablespoon of ajwain in two glasses of water. Once the water boils, reduce the heat and wait until the colour of the water changes to golden brown. Strain and drink the water. Ajwain tea is also given to a woman soon after delivery for five consecutive days for cleansing the system.

Sesame (Thil) seeds have excellent nutritional values. Even though we didn't know all the benefits as we were growing up, our mother used them to make sesame squares and sesame balls both of which were made with roasted sesame seeds and jiggery(molasses). Now we know that they even help in reducing cholesterol

I also remember drinking barley tea water when I had diarrhea. I remember my aunt drinking it for urinary infection. In spite of all the medicinal values of the foods mentioned above, all may not agree with or may not be good for all people. One man's food could be another man's poison. It is very important that patients with medication do not try natural remedies for the same ailments as it could result in overdose. For example; if you are on blood pressure medication, do not take natural remedies which reduce blood pressure, as it may lower your blood pressure too much. Always consult and inform your doctors about any natural remedy you are using.

4

Hot and Cold Foods

When I heard Genevieve aunty talk about hot and cold foods, I remembered what my parents used to say. According to an ancient Ayurvedic science of India, all foods are supposed to be either hot or cool for your body. Ayurvedic medicine, is one of the most ancient medicines of the world. My mother's and grandmother's generation knew these foods well. As I was growing up, I constantly heard my mother say, "That is too heaty or that is cooling to your body."

Ayurveda classifies all human beings into three categories or doshas according to their temperaments and traits. These are Vata, Pitta and Kapha. Each of these categories have foods that are appropriate for them. All I know is that when I was growing up I was called Pitta by my elders and hence was advised to avoid foods that produced heat, as the Pitta people were already hot. You can take a free Dosha quiz on the internet to get a fair idea about your Dosha. Some general guidelines in Ayurveda tell us what foods are good for each Dosha and what foods go together and what foods don't. I only remember some of the things the elders mentioned, such as fruits should always be eaten separately from other foods and ice cold water should be avoided. My mother also said "fruits are gold in the morning, silver at noon and lead at night." As a result we never ate fruits at night. Drinking a glass of buttermilk after food was considered good for health. Most fruits and lentils were said be cooling for your body and most meats and eggs, heaty. Cardamom in coffee is supposed to nullify the bad effects of coffee. In some parts of India, the bride and the groom are given pine nuts to eat the day before their wedding as it is supposed to be an aphrodisiac.

An Ayurvedic doctor can guide and advice a person about what is good for him or her. It was believed that we usually fall sick when the food balance is disturbed. As a result, a person with fever, upset stomach etc. was given foods that were very easy to digest; such as, congee with yogurt and pickle (boiled raw mango or lemon in salt water and vinegar), until they were well again.

Different Foods had to be eaten at different age, condition of your health and time. For example a pregnant woman was supposed to eat foods that were cooling for her body, as it was believed that pregnancy produced more than the needed heat in the body. However, after birth the body became cool because of the loss of blood, fluids and the baby that produced the heat. The body was now cooler than the desired level and therefore to maintain the proper balance, foods that produced heat were given to the mother. There was a special mixture that was given to the mother twice a day. It was prepared with special roots, herbs, garlic, ghee, almonds, etc. and it tasted divine. Non-vegetarians also drank chicken soup made of whole baby chickens for forty days, as chicken is supposed to produce heat.

The mother was given plenty of rest, which includes oil massage for herself and the baby for the forty days following the delivery. A special nurse is often hired to look after the mother and baby. These nurses get good remuneration plus a sari for their services. If people cannot afford a nurse, the women in the family take on the job of looking after the mother and child.

This is what happened in my hometown in the south of India. Customs and traditions vary from state to state in India. The rest that the mother gets and the strength that she gains during those forty days is said to benefit her in coming years. This treatment usually results in the mother and baby looking healthy with their skins glowing and hair shining with new life.

I also remember a cloth being tied very tightly around the mother's stomach after delivery. They said it was done to let the internal organs get back to their original places. This also flattened the mother's stomach. Being the eldest of six children, I have seen it done to my mother. This is an age old custom. I actually used a corset.

I have had the opportunity to watch how babies were bathed. As soon the mother and baby came home from the hospital, they were both massaged daily with coconut oil heated with herbs and then bathed by this special nurse, usually a midwife. The baby was left in a special cradle made from a part of the betel nut tree for an hour with the oil on its body. The nurse or a family member would then exercise the baby by moving its arms and legs and then leave it in this cradle. Every movement of the baby was perceived as its exercise. Then the mother first and then the baby were washed by rubbing a beaten egg first to get rid of the oil and then with baby soap or gram flour. Some babies and mothers might be allergic to gram flour so testing beforehand is extremely important.

Bathing the baby was a production by itself. First, a nurse or midwife would sit on a small flat stool with her sari pulled up very high between her legs and put the baby upside down on her bare stretched legs so that the baby's face fell between her knees and ankles. This gave the baby space to breathe. She then washed the baby's back. Then the baby would be flipped over and washed neck down. The midwife then poured the water with one hand while holding the baby's chin up so as to prevent water from going on the baby's face. After both sides were washed thoroughly, she would wash the baby's face gently. Last to be washed was the baby's head. After gently applying egg, gram flour or soup on the baby's head, she would wash the head.

This was done by placing a stretched hand on the baby's forehead so that it rests snugly between the midwife's thumb and forefinger. This kept the water from entering the baby's eyes, nose or mouth. The baby would be flipped again to wash the back of the head. These women were such experts that it was a pleasure watching. I, being the eldest child, had the opportunity to watch at least four of my siblings being bathed. By the time this ritual of bathing and feeding the baby was over, the baby would be so exhausted that it would sleep for hours before getting up for the next feed. And Mother also got her rest.

A midwife's job was to look after the needs of the mother and baby and to ensure that the mother ate the right food and got enough rest. By the end of those forty days, besides having a healthy glowing skin and hair, the mother and baby also put on quite a bit of weight, which was welcomed and accepted both by the husbands and the society at large in those days. In a country with so much poverty, weight gain was the privilege of the rich. Those days, it was a complement to tell a young woman that she had gained weight, especially after her marriage or birth of her child. It showed that her husband was wealthy and she was happy. The custom is still on.

However, nowadays many new mothers are refusing eat all that rich food prepared just for them and are becoming more active and venturing out before the forty day curfew imposed on the older generation, as weight gain is no more in fashion.

5

Natural Beauty Treatments

Genevieve aunty was not as familiar with the various beauty treatments we used in India as I was. Girls of her generation were not into these things as much as our generation was. Most of our beauty treatments when I was growing up were home made. But remember to test for allergy on a small part of your hand or face before using any facial masks or homemade mixtures.

Honey:

Honey is excellent for blemishes. Heat honey slightly and spread over the face. Leave for 5 to 10 minutes and wash off. Honey is said to tighten and brighten the skin. Honey has antiseptic qualities as well. Honey mixed with gram flower and lemon juice used as a mask is excellent for skin problems such as marks from Acne. However, some are allergic to gram flour and therefore should test the skin with a tiny bit at first and wait until it dries and wash off to see if there is any reaction. It is also not advisable for very dry skin types. Honey mixed with white of an egg and gram flour is also good for acne. This too should be tried on a small part of the face before applying to test for allergy. Honey should not be used on eyebrows, lashes and hair as it is believed that it can grey the hair.(You don't want white eyebrows and lashes.)

Fruit:

Many fruits have good ingredients beneficial for the skin. When you eat a fruit, rub some of it gently on your face and wash it off when it dries.

Eggs:

When you make eggs for breakfast, whatever egg white that remains in the shell should go on your face, unless you have very dry skin. It is excellent for normal and oily skin. Wash it off when it is dry. The results will be amazing within a week.

Glycerine:

Glycerine mixed with rosewater and lemon is excellent to prevent wrinkles. It also softens and lightens any black marks on the skin. Glycerine and Vaseline is the best cure for rough heels. Wash your feet thoroughly, dry them and apply the mixture of Vaseline and glycerine. Wear socks while you sleep.

True Story:

When I was living in a women's hostel in Bombay, my friends and I had a competition as to who would have the best looking feet in two weeks. Every night after washing our feet we applied a mixture of glycerine, lemon juice and Vaseline, then wore socks and went to bed. Next morning we washed our feet thoroughly with soap and a brush, because India is very dusty except during the rainy season and women wear open shoes or sandals. The results in two weeks were unbelievable. Our feet looked beautiful with such soft heals that we could not decide whose feet looked the best. A pedicure after that just enhanced the look.

Coconut Juice and Oil:

Coconut oil and juice are both excellent for black spots on the face or body and also give a glow to your skin. Coconut oil is also excellent for hair.

True story:

I still remember my little cousin who had some rash on his face and was left with visible black spots. He being light skinned, the marks were very conspicuous. All my aunt did was, apply freshly squeezed coconut juice on his face every day. By the end of my holiday of a month with them, his face was completely cleared of the marks.

Face Masks:

It is always important to see if you are allergic to something if you have never used it before, by applying a little on the corner of your face and looking for any reaction. We used a lot of face masks during our college days. Sandalwood was considered to be the best. Since sandalwood like Neem and turmeric is very potent and can burn the skin, these have to be used in very small proportions (a pinch or two). You need to wash your face thoroughly and if possible steam and remove blackheads before applying the mask. Keep the mask on until it is dry and then wash it off. Do not talk while the mask is on.

Here are some suggested recipes for face masks:

Milk or yogurt: 1 spoon
Sandalwood powder: 1/8 teaspoon
Turmeric only a pinch
Powdered oatmeal or 'Fuller's Earth' (enough to make a thick paste.)
Honey 1/2 teaspoon

Mix it with yogurt or any fruit juice or pureed fruit to make a thick paste. Fuller's Earth can be used with any fruit juice to make simple face masks. The Indian name for 'Fuller's Earth' is 'Multani Mutti.' Milk cream and egg white mixture is good for older skin. People with oily skin should avoid oils, yolk of an egg, and honey in their face pack. People with dry skin should avoid lemon juice and white of an egg in their face pack. Papaya is supposed to have pectin and antacids to cleanse and brighten the skin. Therefore it is an excellent ingredient to use in masks or by itself.

Home Remedies for Dandruff:

Coconut oil: 2 tablespoons
Lemon Juice: 1 tablespoon

Massage your scalp with this mixture, leave it for four hours and then shampoo or wash with Sikakai powder. The botanical name for Shikakai is, Acacia Concinna. Cut lime into half, dip it in salt and massage it on your scalp and leave it for 1/2 an hour and wash it off. Massage the scalp with yogurt that is left out of the fridge for three days. Leave it for 1/2 an hour and wash it off with some mild shampoo or shikakai powder.

Remedy for falling hair:

Massaging your scalp with coconut oil which has been boiled with shikakai and Amla (gooseberry). It is excellent for hair loss. Coconut milk is also beneficial for falling hair. Ayurveda gives a lot of importance to Amla (gooseberry), in the maintenance and improvement of the texture and growth of hair.

Acne:

Don't forget to test for allergy, first. Dandruff and bad stomach can be two of the causes for acne and pimples. Therefore it is very important to get rid of your dandruff, keep your skin clean by washing it with a mixture of 'Multani Mutti' or 'Fuller's Earth' and rosewater. Eating lots of fruits and vegetables and avoiding fried food is good. Cleaning the face with lemon and oatmeal powder is better than soap. A face pack of bran, baking soda and water is good for acne skin. Make a paste of yogurt and ground ajwain or carom seeds and apply it on the face for acne or pimples.

Eyes:

Cucumber slices are placed on the eye for fifteen minutes before going for a party to brighten the eyes and lessen the appearance of black circles around the eye. However, black circles can be caused by lack of sleep, stress, eye strain, constipation and hereditary factors. It is therefore very important to get proper sleep and take care of the stomach as well.

Hair Growth:

Castor oil is excellent for hair growth. When girls have very thin eyelashes or eyebrows, castor oil is applied. Kajal or homemade eyeliner, paste of sandalwood and turmeric to get rid of facial hair, using hydrogen peroxide to make dark facial hair less conspicuous was part of our beauty regimen. But do not use this if you have never used it before. It might burn your skin.

Hair Removal:

Kajal: Place a plate over two small containers of about 4" high. Light a diya or clay lamp with castor oil in it and place it below the plate for about 20 minutes. You will see black soot accumulated at the bottom of the plate. Carefully collect this black powder in a stainless steel box with a blunt knife. Mix this powder with a few drops of castor oil. It is now ready to use. It has to be made under proper hygienic conditions in order to be used. Rub a stick of sandalwood on a grinding stone with half a teaspoon of milk until you get some of the wood mixed into the milk. You can see the colour change. Now rub a piece of the turmeric root on to the mixture. When the mixture thickens, use it on your face where there is facial hair. Wait for it to dry and then rub gently with the pumice stone. The hair will come out with the mask.

> Caution: Test for burning and any reaction, first.
> Wash the mask off the minute it starts burning.
> Be gentle with the pumice stone.

6

Vegetarian Recipes

"It is my view that the vegetarian manner of living, by its purely physical effect on the human temperament, would most beneficially influence the lot of mankind."

—Albert Einstein

A list of very good foods:

Yogurt, plain
Sweet potato
Kiwi
All berries
Butternut squash
Broccoli
Avocado
Peas
Flaxseed
Kale
Multigrain crackers and breads
Edamame or green soybean
Lentils
Quinoa
Fish oil
Cooked tomatoes
Cherry tomatoes
Ginger and garlic eaten raw or used in cooking
Onions sautéed
Multigrain bread and crackers
Bananas: 1/2 a day if it is big
Mixture of honey and cinnamon powder eaten on breads or boiled in water and drunk as tea
Sprouted lentils or beans eaten raw or used in soups and stir fry

Try to use less salt in all your food to remain healthy and in order to keep your blood pressure under control.

Porridge (We drank this when we were kids.):

Equal amount of Finger Millet and Wheat

Wash and soak both of the above grains separately for a day.

Drain the water, wash once more, drain and then tie the grains separately in a cheese cloth and hang it where there is some sunlight.

By evening you will see some sprouts.

Sprinkle about three tablespoons of water on the cheese cloth and keep for another day. You will see more sprouts.

Dry the sprouted grains in the sun for about four days or until the grains are dry with no moisture.

Grind separately and then mix and keep in a airtight container

Take two tablespoons of this porridge mixture and with little water make it into a paste

See that there are no granules.

Now mix 2 cups of water and 2 cups of milk, a little at a time to avoid any granules.

Cook on a low flame until the porridge is well cooked to the consistency you want.

Add a little honey for taste and drink a glass if it is thin or eat a bowlful if it is thick.

Soups

Vegetable soup

Cut 2 or 21/2 cups of vegetables of your choice into small pieces and boil them in water for 15 minutes. (celery, Carrots, peas, green beans and tomatoes are good) Carrot could be cut into thin slices. Avoid potatoes Don't forget to add finely chopped garlic and ginger to the soup with the vegetables. Add dill, parsley or coriander according to your preference with finely chopped green onion just 5 minutes before turning the heat off. Add salt and pepper to taste. If you want the soup thick, boil 2 carrots and a tomato separately and grind them and add to the soup. If you like a bit of zinc to your soup, add a green chilly finely cut with the vegetables. Cook multigrain pasta or quinoa separately and add to the soup. Then it becomes a meal by itself.

Carrot and Tomato Soup with Coriander Ingredients

> Water: about 26 ounces
> Carrots: 3 peeled and cut into cubes
> Tomatoes: 3 with skin and seeds removed
> Onion: 1
> Garlic: 4 cloves
> Coriander: 1/2 cup washed and finely chopped
> Salt and pepper to taste
> Milk: 1/2 cup

Boil all the ingredients except coriander until they are properly cooked. Blend in a blender. Add chopped coriander. Bring the soup to a boil and lower the heat. Add milk and stir. Add pepper and salt to taste.

Lentil and Vegetable Soup

> Lentils: 1/2 cup
> Onion: 1 large chopped
> Carrots: 2 cleaned and grated
> Green beans: 1/2 cup chopped
> Tomato: 1 finely chopped (remove seeds and skin)
> Celery: 2 cups finely chopped
> Coriander: handful washed and chopped finely
> Garlic: 6 pods finely chopped
> Green Chilly: 1 finely chopped
> Apple cider vinegar: 1 teaspoon
> Salt to taste
> Asafoetida: 1/4 teaspoon (to prevent gas)

Soak lentils overnight. Wash in the morning and add fresh water (about 6 to 7 cups).

Boil the lentils first. When they are almost done, add the vegetables except coriander. Boil until the vegetables are tender. Add water as per your desired consistency. Add the vinegar and salt to taste and garnish with finely chopped coriander leaves and asafoetida.

A bowl of this soup with a slice of multigrain bread is a good meal.

Sweet corn and Egg Soup (Omit the egg if you do not eat eggs)

> Sweet corn: 2 cans (buy the one with the least sodium)
> Egg: 1 well beaten
> Apple cider vinegar: 1 teaspoon
> Green onion: 1/4 cup finely chopped
> Salt and pepper to taste

Empty the cans of sweet corn in a pot with a cup of water and let it boil. Stir occasionally. Add water if necessary.

When the corn is boiling, add the beaten egg and stir with a fork. You will see strands of egg forming in the soup.

Now add vinegar and finely chopped green onions. Switch the stove off. Add salt if required.

Moong Dhal (Split Lotus seeds) and Green onion soup

Half cup of moong dhal soaked overnight
1 green chilli
1 tomato with skin and seeds removed
3 cloves of garlic
A piece of ginger
1 bunch of green onion finely chopped
Salt to taste
1 tablespoon of apple cider vinegar

Wash the soaked dhal twice and boil it with 3 to 4 cups of water.

Once the mixture boils, lower the heat to almost minimum, close the lid and let it simmer for about 15 minutes or until the dhal is done.

Check after every 5 minutes to see if there is enough water.

Once the dhal is done, add rest of the ingredients except the vinegar and green onions and cook for another 6 minutes.

Grind all the ingredients in a blender and pour the mixture back into the pot.

Add the vinegar and chopped green onion stir, close the lid and let stand. Add water according to the consistency you want and salt to taste.

The soup is ready to eat.

Rice Dishes

Since I have been introduced to quinoa, I have been substituting rice with quinoa. You can cook quinoa the same way as you cook rice. Even though, basmati rice is very aromatic and tasty, it is full of carbohydrates that will turn into sugar. Therefore, it is better to consume it in small quantities and occasionally. Brown rice is a better substitute.

Plain Basmati Rice

> Basmati rice: 1 cup
> Water: 2 cups
> Olive oil or butter: 1 tablespoon
> Lemon juice of 1/2 a lemon
> Salt: 1/2 teaspoon
> Cardamom: 2
> Cinnamon stick: 1 inch long

Wash rice at least three times and drain.

Heat the oil or butter in a pot and fry the cinnamon and cardamom for 1 or 2 minutes on medium heat.

Add drained rice and fry for another two minutes.

Add water, salt and lemon juice and raise the heat to high and wait until the water boils.

Lower the heat to minimum, close the pot and let it cook for 10 to 12 minutes.

Shut of the heat, let it stand for 5 minutes and fluff the rice with a fork.

Cabbage and Carrot rice with almonds

> Rice: 2 cups
> Cabbage finely chopped: 1 cup
> Carrots grated: 1 cup
> Almonds cut or sliced: 1/4 cup
> Cinnamon stick: 1" long
> Cardamoms: 2
> Cloves: 3
> Salt: 3/4 teaspoon
> A pinch of turmeric powder or saffron for colour
> Butter or olive oil: 2 tablespoons
> Juice of 1 lemon
> Water: 4 1/2 cups

Wash the rice at least three times and drain.

Fry the cinnamon, cardamom and cloves in oil or butter on medium heat for one or two minutes.

Add the almonds and fry them for another 2/3 minutes: light brown.

Add the cabbage and carrots and fry for 5 minutes stirring regularly.

Add the rice and lemon juice and continue to fry for 3 minutes.

Add water and salt, turn the heat to high and wait until it boils.

Turn the heat to minimum, close the pot and let it cook for 10-12 minutes.

Switch the stove off and let it stand for 5 more minutes and then fluff it with a fork.

You can replace cabbage and carrots with mixed vegetables.

Coriander Rice

Rice: 2 cups
Water: 3 cups
Salt: 1/2 teaspoon
Butter/Olive oil: 1 tablespoon
Cloves: 2
Cinnamon stick: 2 inches long
Cardamoms: 2
Coriander: 1 cup very finely chopped
Juice of 1 lemon

Wash and drain the rice and set aside.

Melt butter or oil in a pot and add cinnamon, cardamoms and cloves and stir on low heat for 2 to 3 minutes.

Add rice and stir for 5 minutes on medium heat.

Add coriander, salt, lemon juice and water and bring it to a boil.

Turn the heat on low and cook for 10 to 12 minutes.

Switch the stove off and let stand for 5 more minutes.

Open the pot and fluff the rice wit a fork.

Serve as a side dish.

Dill and Parsley Rice (Irani style)

Basmati Rice: 1 cup
Water: 1 1/2 cups
Dill: 1 bunch cleaned without stems and finely chopped
Parsley: 1/2 a bunch cleaned without stems and finely chopped
Potatoes: 2 washed and sliced
Pitted sour cherries or dried cranberries: 1 cup
Cloves: 3, Cardamom: 2, Cinnamon sticks: 2 (inch long)
Frozen lima or soya beans: 1 cup
Olive oil: 4 tablespoons
Salt to taste

Wash the rice thoroughly.

Heat olive oil in a non stick pot on medium heat. Add cinnamon sticks, cardamom and cloves and fry for two minutes or until you get the aroma.

Add rice and stir for two minutes. Add water and salt.

Stir and wait for the water to come to a boil.

Close the pot with a lid and lower the heat to minimum (about 10 minutes).

Cook until the water is absorbed. Rice will not be fully cooked. Set the rice aside.

In another non stick pot, heat the other 2 tablespoons of oil.

Place the sliced potatoes at the bottom.

Then place one layer of rice, one layer of chopped dill and parsley and some frozen lima beans topped with sour cherries/cranberries

Repeat this until all the rice, herbs, lima beans and cherries are over.

Close the lid and cook this for 45 to 50 minutes on a medium to low heat.

The potatoes at the bottom will become crisp when the rice is done.

Empty the whole pot of rice on a platter

Arrange the crispy potato slices on the side.

Khichdi (Rice with Dahls and vegetables)

Basmati rice washed and soaked in water: 2 cups
Water: 4 1/2 cups
Washed and soaked moong dahl (lotus seed): 1/4 cup
Washed and soaked masur dahl (split lentil): 1/4 cup
Chopped onions: 4
Peas: 1 cup
Minced garlic 1/2 tablespoon
Minced ginger: 1/2 tablespoon
Green chilly chopped: 1
Turmeric powder: 1/2 tablespoon
Garam Masala: 1 tablespoon
Chilli Powder: 1/2 teaspoon
Chopped coriander: 1/2 cup
Olive oil: 2 tablespoons
Salt to taste
Juice of 1 lemon

Fry the chopped onions in olive oil until they are light brown on medium heat.

Add ginger, garlic, green chilli and continue to fry for another 3 minutes on low heat.

Add Garam Masala, chilli powder, turmeric powder and fry for another minute.

Drain the dahls and add them to the mixture and fry for another 2 minutes.

Add 4 cups of water bring the mixture to a boil and let the dahls cook for 5 minutes on low heat.

Add rice and another half cup of water, coriander, lemon juice and salt and bring it to a boil.

As soon as the mixture boils, stir the mixture and lower the heat to minimum and let it cook for 10-12 minutes (cover the pot).

Open the lid, fluff the rice and serve with yogurt or cudy.

Cudy

Chickpea flour: 2 tablespoons
Water: 2 cups
Yogurt plain stirred: 1 cup
Green chilly sliced into half: 1
Ginger finely sliced: 1 inch piece
Lemon juice: 2 tablespoons
Brown sugar: heaped tablespoon
Salt: very little
Turmeric: 1/4 teaspoon
Oil: 2 tablespoons
Cumin seeds: 1/2 teaspoon
Curry Leaves: 1 teaspoon
Dry Red chilli: 1
Fresh coriander chopped: 1/2 cup

Mix the chickpea flour in 3 tablespoons of water to form a thick paste without any granules.

Add the rest of the water, turmeric powder, green chilli, lemon juice and ginger and cook on medium heat stirring constantly for about 10 to 15 minutes.

Turn the heat to low and add yogurt, salt, lemon juice and sugar and bring it gradually to a boil. Switch off the heat and put it aside.

Heat the oil on medium heat and when it is hot, put the cumin seeds, curry leaves and red chilly in it. Cover the pan and wait until the sound of popping cumin seeds stop, and then pour it on the cudy.

Garnish with chopped fresh coriander.

Khichdi and cudy are eaten the day after a very heavy meal.

Healthy Salad

Lettuce: 1 head, shredded
Chick peas: 1/2 cup
Orange wedges: 1 can
Apples: 2 peeled and sliced
Walnuts: 1/2 cup
Cucumber: 1 peeled and sliced
Tomato: 1 (cut into 8 pieces)
Broccoli: 1 cup (cut into medium size pieces)

Dressing:

Mix 2 1/2 spoons of olive oil, 2 spoons of balsamic vinegar, a dash of pepper and 1 teaspoon of honey and mix well. You can substitute honey with pureed strawberries or raspberries.
Pour the dressing on the salad mix and serve.

Quinoa or Cuscus Salad with Vegetables and Almonds

Blanched roasted almonds: 1/4 cup
Olive oil: 3/4 cup
Balsamic vinegar: 4 tablespoons
Mixed vegetables boiled (not too soft): 1 cup
Chopped thyme: 1 tablespoon
Couscous: 1 1/2 cup
Water: 1 1/4 cup

Or

Quinoa: 1 cup
Water: 2 cups
Pepper: 1/2 teaspoon
Salt: 1/4 teaspoon

Mix thyme, salt, pepper, vinegar and oil and set aside.

Bring the water to a boil and add the couscous and stir well.

Remove the pan from the fire and let it stand for 5 minutes.

If you are using quinoa, cook quinoa separately with a ratio of 1 to 2 (1cup quinoa to 2 cups of water).

Cook mixed vegetables with 1/4 cup water on a low to medium heat until they are almost done. Close the lid and set aside for 5 minutes.

In a large bowl mix the couscous or quinoa, vegetables, almonds and the dressing.

Raita (yogurt salad)

Plain yogurt 2%: 2 cups
Cucumber: 1 large
Salt: 1/2 tablespoon
Paprika: a pinch
Pepper: a pinch
Coriander: 1/4 cup finely chopped
Green chilly: 1 finely chopped
Brown sugar: 1/2 teaspoon

Wash, peel and grate the cucumber, mix it with salt and set aside for 5 minutes.

Squeeze the water from the grated cucumber and mix the cucumber well with yogurt and the rest of the ingredients. Throw out the squeezed water.

You may add nuts, chopped tomato and carrot if you so desire. You can use Raita with any kind of rice

Chickpea Salad

Chickpeas: 1 can
Onions: 2
Green chillies: 1 or 2
Coriander: 1/2 bunch
Apple cider vinegar: 3 tablespoons
Olive oil: 2 tablespoons

Chop onions and green chillies finely and soak them in vinegar for 20 minutes.

Wash and drain the chickpeas and mix them with the rest of the ingredients. No salt is necessary as the chickpeas already have salt.

7

Dahl or Lentils and Vegetable Dishes
(Tur Dahl, Masoor Dahl, Moong Dahl, Chana Dahl, Udath Dahl)

*Y*ou can get the ingredients for these recipes at Indian grocery stores. You can use one type or have a mixture of two or more.

Dhal

Udath Dhal: 1 cup
Onion: 1 finely chopped
Lemon: 1
Garlic: 4 cloves: finely chopped
Ginger: grated, 1 teaspoon
Green chillies: 2 cut vertically into two
Tomato: 1 finely chopped
Turmeric powder: a pinch
Olive oil: 2 teaspoons
Coriander: 1/2 cup chopped finely
Salt: 1/2 teaspoon

Wash and soak dhal overnight.

Wash it three times with clean water the next morning and cook it with 3 cups of water, salt and turmeric(high until the water boils and then on low and covered until the dhal is cooked).

Throw the fin that comes on the top.

Mash the dhal with a ladle and set aside.

Fry the onion, garlic, ginger and green chillies in olive oil for 10 minutes on medium to low heat.

Add tomatoes and fry for another 10 minutes.

Add the dhal and lemon juice and bring it to a boil, stirring constantly so that the dhal does not stick to the bottom.

Garnish with chopped coriander.

Serve it with plain basmati rice or roti/nan/pita P.S.: You may add green peppers, cauliflower or spinach to make it more wholesome.

Pan Fried Sweet Potato, Egg Plant and Potato with Chickpea Flour

Vegetables: any 2 of the above
Chickpea flour: 1 cup
Water :1/2 cup
Chilly powder: 1/4 teaspoon
Salt: 1/4 teaspoon
Olive oil: enough to grease the non-stick pan

Wash and peel the skin off the vegetables.

Cut them into thin slices and set aside.

Mix the chickpea flour, salt, chilly powder and water to make a thick paste, rather messy (It may be too thick to dip the vegetables in it).

Apply the paste on both sides of the sliced vegetables and place them on a heated non-stick pan. Fry both sides on medium heat until done.

Left over Rice Bajias

Left over rice: 1 cup
Coriander: 1/4 cup finely chopped
Green chilly: 1 finely chopped
Onion: 1 finely chopped
Chick pea flour: 3-4 tablespoons
Salt to taste

Wash your hands well and mix all the above ingredients until the mixture becomes sticky and messy. The water from the onions, coriander and green chillies will be enough for the mixture.

Clean your hands off the mixture with a spoon.

Wash your hands and form flat rounds from the mixture with wet hands and set them aside on a foil.

You will have to wet your hands often, so that the mixture does not stick to your hands.

Fry them on a non-stick pan until both sides are done (Medium to low heat).

Use these as starters or Hors D'oeuvres.

Spinach and Cheese (Paneer)
(You get Paneer in any Indian grocery store)

> Frozen cut spinach packets: 2
> Paneer: slab
> Ginger: grated: 1 tablespoon
> Tomatoes skinned and chopped finely: 2
> Cumin seed roasted and crushed: 1 teaspoon
> Chilli powder to taste: (1/4 to 1/2 teaspoon)
> Salt to taste: 1/4 teaspoon
> Olive oil 2 tablespoons
> Half a lemon

Boil the frozen spinach in its own water for 10 minutes.

Grind it in the blender and set aside.

In a pan heat oil and fry the ginger and cumin powder for 5 minutes on low heat.

Add chopped tomatoes and chilli powder and continue to fry until the mixture becomes homogenous.

Add the ground spinach, lemon and salt and bring it to a boil on medium heat and set aside

Cut the paneer into rectangular pieces (2"x1"x1").

Fry them to golden brown on low heat on a non-stick pan with minimum oil.

Add the paneer to the spinach. Add more salt if necessary.

Sweet Potatoes/Cauliflower/Peas

Cauliflower: 1 small
Sweet Potatoes: 2 medium
Peas: 1 cup
Water: 1 cup
Cumin powder: 1/4 teaspoon
Coriander powder: 1/2 teaspoon
Chilly powder: 1/4 teaspoon
Turmeric powder: 1/8 teaspoon
Onion: 1 (chopped finely)
Tomatoes: 2 (skinned and chopped finely)
Fresh coriander: 1/2 cup finely chopped

Wash and cut the sweet potatoes, and cauliflower into pieces (size of potato salad).

Boil the potatoes in half a cup of water on low heat (covered) until the potatoes are almost done (add more water if needed).

Add cauliflower and peas and cook for another 6-7 minutes.

In a pan heat oil and fry the chopped onions until they are light brown.

Add the powdered spices and fry for 2 more minutes.

Add chopped tomatoes and fry for 5 more minutes.

Add the boiled vegetables, bring it to a boil and garnish with chopped coriander.

Eggplant slices with yogurt

Egg plant: 1 large
Yogurt plain 2%: 500 gm (17.637 oz)
Paprika: dash
Pepper: dash
Red chilli powder: pinch
Salt: 1/8 teaspoon
Olive oil: 1 tablespoon

Brown sugar: 1 teaspoon

Make the yogurt mixture by mixing yogurt with salt and sugar and set aside.

Wash and cut egg plant into thin slices, apply a mixture of chilli powder, salt and a little pepper and pan fry on a non stick pan flipping sides for 4 minutes on each side.

Arrange them on a semi flat bowl cover with foil and keep them warm in the oven at minimum heat.

Pour the yogurt mixture evenly on the slices, just before serving.

Garnish with a dash of paprika and pepper (chopped coriander is optional).

Vegetable Patties

Boiled and mashed sweet potatoes: 2
Carrot grated: 1
A piece of cabbage finely chopped
Green peas: 1/2 cup
Green beans finely chopped: 1/2 cup
Onion finely chopped: 1
Coriander finely chopped: 1/2 bunch
Green chillies finely chopped: 2 long
Egg (white): 1
Breadcrumbs or cream of wheat: 1 cup
Olive oil: 2 tablespoons
Lemon Juice: 1 tablespoon
Salt to taste
bread crumbs: 1/4 cup

In a pan, fry all the onion and green chillies until the onions are light brown with 2 tablespoons of oil.

Stir fry until the vegetables are almost cooked and turn off stove.

Add the mashed sweet potatoes and coriander and set aside.

Add salt and bread crumbs.

When warm enough to handle, shape them into patties and set aside.

Beat the white of an egg with a pinch of salt.

Apply egg mixture to each patty and then roll each in the breadcrumbs.

Place carefully on the non-stick pan which should be ready on the stove.

Fry patties on medium heat until each side is brown (5 to 8 minutes).

Turn the sides and fry for another five minutes.

The patties are ready to serve.

8

Non Vegetarian Dishes

*I*f you want broth, boil 4 chicken thighs and legs in a large skillet of water with a piece of crushed ginger, two finely cut onions and 5 to 7 cloves of crushed garlic for about 45 minutes. Once the water boils turn the heat to medium. Strain the liquid and store the broth. Instead of chicken, you can use lean veal or beef for broth. Once you have the base, half your work is done. You can shred the chicken into the soup. Freeze part of this broth. Add the vegetables that you like and whole grain pasta or quinoa if you wish and you have a good sumptuous soup. Add salt and pepper according to your taste.

Lentil and Sausage soup

> Lentils: 1/2 cup
> Onion: 1 large chopped
> Carrots: 2 cleaned and grated
> Green beans: 1/2 cup chopped
> Tomato: 1 finely chopped
> Celery: 2 cups finely chopped
> Coriander: handful washed and chopped finely
> Garlic: 6 pods finely chopped
> Green Chilly: 1 finely chopped
> Hot Italian sausages: 5
> Apple cider vinegar: 1 teaspoon
> Salt to taste

Boil Sausages in water until they all float on the top of the pot. Turn off the heat and let it cool.

Cut them into 1" long pieces and set aside.

Soak lentils overnight. Wash in the morning and add fresh water (about 6 to 7 cups).

Boil the lentils with all the vegetables except coriander until they are tender.

Add the sausages and coriander and give it a boil. Add water as per your desired consistency.

Add the vinegar and salt. A bowl of this soup with a multigrain slice of bread is a good meal.

Sweet corn, chicken and egg soup

Sweet corn: 2 cans (buy the one with the least sodium
Egg: 1 well beaten
Apple cider vinegar: 1 teaspoon
Breast of chicken: 1 boneless and skinless cut into tiny pieces.
Green onion: 1/4 cup finely chopped
Salt and pepper to taste

Empty the cans of sweet corn in a pot with a cup of water and let it come to a boil add the chicken and let it cook on medium heat. Don't forget to stir often when the soup is boiling, add the beaten egg and stir lightly until you see the strings of egg in the soup.

Add vinegar and finely chopped green onions.

Switch the stove off. Add salt if required.

It is always a good idea to use less salt in your food.

Chicken, Beef or Veal soup

Chicken leg quarters skinned (beef or veal bones): 2
Green onion finely chopped: 1
Garlic finely chopped: 2 pods
Ginger grated: 1 tiny piece
Dill finely chopped: handfull

Tomato skinned and seeded and chopped
Salt and pepper to taste
Apple cider vinegar: 1 tablespoon

Boil the chicken, beef or veal in 5 cups of water (bring it to a boil then lower the heat to medium) for 15 minutes.
Remove the chicken from the broth and cut into cubes.
Strain the broth and add all the other ingredients except dill.
Boil for about 15 more minutes on medium heat.
Add the chicken and dill stir well and the soup is ready

Chicken Salad

Chicken breasts: 2 skinless-boneless
Lettuce: 1 head
Bread croutons: 1 cup
Use the Vinegar/olive oil/honey/pepper dressing (1 tablespoon of each and 2 pinches of pepper)
Salt
Lemon juice: 1/2 juicy lemon
Walnuts: 1/2 cup

Marinate chicken breast with salt, pepper and lemon juice for twenty minutes and bake in a preheated oven (350 degrees) for 20 minutes on either side.
Cut the chicken into pieces (2" x 1/2").
Shred the lettuce and mix it with chicken, walnuts and salad dressing.
Ready to serve.

Tuna or Salmon Salad

Tuna or Salmon: 1 can
Pickle: 1
Celery: 1 cup
Apple cider vinegar: 1 tablespoon

Olive oil: 3/4 tablespoon
Green chilli: 1 finely chopped (optional)
Red onion: 1/2 finely chopped
Salt (only if needed, as there is salt in the pickle and tuna)

Mix the green chilli and onion in vinegar and let it stand for 15 minutes.
Drain the water from tuna and flake it.
Mix all the ingredients.

Chicken in Yogurt

Chicken: 1 kg (2 lb, 3.274 oz)
Garlic ginger paste: 2 tablespoons
Paprika: 1 tablespoon
Olive oil: 1 tablespoon
Onion: 1
Lemon: 1
Salt to taste
Yogurt 2 or 3%: 1 cup
Cardamom: 2
Cloves: 3
Cinnamon stick: 2" long

Ginger Garlic Paste

Grind 1 cup of peeled garlic, 1 cup of ginger (scraped and cut into cubs) and apple cider vinegar (enough for the blender to work). Store it in a bottle in the fridge and use it when necessary. You can even use some green chillies in the mixture. It is good for months.

Skin the chicken. If it is a whole chicken skin, wash and cut.
Put 1" cuts on the pieces, squeeze the lemon on it and set aside.
Cut and fry the onion in olive oil until it turns light brown.
Add cardamom, cinnamon and cloves and fry for another 2 minutes.

Put the chicken in the same pot and fry on medium heat for 5 minutes.

Add the ginger garlic paste, paprika and salt and let it cook for about 25 minutes stirring often on medium heat.

Lower the heat to minimum and add yogurt. Mix well, taste, add salt if needed.

Continue to cook for 2 more minutes.

Serve with Basmati rice or nan.

Green Chicken Curry

Chicken: 1 kg (2 lb, 3.274 oz)
Potatoes: 2 medium
Coriander: 1 bunch
Onions: 2 large
Tomatoes:3 (seeded and skinned)
Cinnamon: 1" long
Cardamoms: 2
Olive oil: 2 tablespoons
Cloves: 3
Green chillies: 4 (medium spicy)
Lemon juice of I lemon
Salt to taste

Skin the chicken. If it is whole, skin and cut it into medium pieces. Put 1" cuts on each piece, mix the lemon juice and set aside.

Cut and fry the onions until golden brown add tomatoes and cook for another 3 minutes.

Grind it with the coriander, chillies and 1 cardamom, 1 clove and half of the cinnamon stick.

Heat the oil and fry the remaining cardamom, cloves and cinnamon stick for 2 minutes on medium heat. Mix the chicken, potatoes, salt and the ground spices and cook on medium heat for 15 minutes stirring occasionally.

Lower the heat and add water (1/4 or 1/2 cup) according to your desired consistency and cook for another 20 minutes.

Add water only if necessary, taste and add salt if needed.
Enjoy with Basmati rice or nan.

The same recipe can be used for veal or mutton. Mutton needs to be cooked 20 minutes on medium heat and 30 minutes on low heat (may need more water)

Chicken or Mutton Biriyani

Prepare the green chicken or mutton curry with not more than 2 cups of gravy. Remember to cook mutton longer than chicken.

Wash and boil 1 1/2 cups of rice with lots of water until it is half done and then drain the water.

Pour the chicken or mutton curry into an ovenware pan (12" x 8"). Slightly larger or smaller dimensions will not harm.

Spread the drained rice evenly on the top of the curry and bake in the preheated oven (350°) for 15 minutes

Serve it with Raita.

If you want vegetable biryani, use cauliflower, peas, potatoes and cashew nuts instead of chicken or mutton, eat this with Raita (Yogurt Salad).

Chicken Wrap

Boneless chicken breasts: 4 (cut into strips)
Paprika powder: 1/4 teaspoon
Ginger garlic paste: 1 1/2 teaspoon
Salt: 1/4 teaspoon
Olive oil: 1 teaspoon

Marinate the chicken strips with the above ingredients for 1/2 an hour and bake in a pre-heated oven (350°) for 20 minutes.

Serve it with chopped lettuce, tomatoes, pickle, grated cheese and hot peppers (optional), wrapped in a whole wheat chapatti or tortilla.

Lean beef/chicken/ burgers

Lean ground beef/chicken/veal: 1 kg (2 lb, 3.274 oz)
Onion: 1 finely chopped
Coriander: 1/2 cup finely chopped
Ginger/garlic paste: 1 tablespoon
Egg: 1 beaten
Bread crumbs: 1/4 cup
Salt: 1/2 teaspoon

Mix all ingredients in a large bowl.
Form into burgers.
Bake in the oven for 20 minutes each side.

Roast Chicken

Chicken: 1 medium
Olive Oil: 1 tablespoon
Vinegar: 1 tablespoon
Chilli powder: 1/2 teaspoon
Crushed garlic and ginger: 1 tablespoon
Paprika: 1 teaspoon
Pepper powder: 1/2 teaspoon
Salt: 1/4 teaspoon
Potatoes: 2
Carrots: 2

Peal and cut the potatoes and carrots and set aside.

Wash, put cuts on the chicken and marinate it with the above spices and salt for 1 hour.

Place the chicken in the centre of the baking dish. Spread the vegetables around and bake for 30 minutes on each side in the preheated oven (350 degrees).

Serve with brown bread and salad (use the meat thermometer to make sure that the chicken is well done.

Butter Chicken

Chicken: 500 gm (17.637 oz)
Butter: 3 tablespoons
Ginger/garlic paste: 1 1/2 tablespoons
Cinnamon powder: 1/4 teaspoon
Chilly Powder: 1 teaspoon
Coriander Powder: 1 tablespoon
Ground Cashew or almonds: 3 tablespoons
Turmeric Powder: 1/4 teaspoon
Tomato paste: 2 tablespoons
Yogurt 2%: 1/2 cup

Wash and cut the chicken into small cubes mix it with the ginger garlic paste and set aside.

Melt butter in a large pan and fry the onions to golden brown on medium heat.

Add powdered spices and continue to fry for another minute.

Add the chicken and cook stirring constantly until the chicken turns white.

Add the tomato paste and ground cashew or almonds and mix thoroughly.

Cook on medium to low heat for 30/35 minutes.

Add stirred yogurt and mix well.

Turn off heat.

Serve with plain basmati rice.

Crispy Healthy Chicken

Chicken: boneless, skinless cut in strips
Wheat thins: 1 1/2 cups finely crushed
Chilly powder 1/4 teaspoon
Mustard: 1/2 teaspoon
Milk: 1/2 cup
Salt: 1/2 teaspoon

Preheat oven at 300 degrees.
Line baking sheet with buttered foil.

Mix milk with mustard, salt and chilli powder.

Place wheat thin crumbs in another plate or shallow dish.

Dip each chicken strip first in the milk mixture and then in the cracker crumbs and bake for 15 minutes on either side Dip: Mix 1 cup of 3% yogurt with juice of 1/2 lemon and a pinch of salt and paprika.

Chicken Stir Fry

Chicken breasts: 2 washed and cut into thin strips 2" long
Green pepper cut into thin strips: 1
Red Pepper cut into thin strips: 1
Green beans cut into strips: 1/2 cup
Green onion cut 1" long: 2 bunches
Mushrooms: 1/4 cup
Carrots cut flat 2" long: 2
Ginger finely grated: 1" piece
Green chilli: 1 cut finely
Soya sauce: 1 1/2 tablespoons
Salt or fried rice seasoning: 1/4 teaspoon
Chilli sauce: 1/2 teaspoon (optional)
Lemon juice: 1 tablespoon
Olive oil: 1 tablespoon
Corn flour: 1 flat teaspoon

Marinate the chicken strips in soya sauce, chilli sauce, lemon juice and salt and set aside.

Heat the olive oil in a wok and fry the grated ginger and green chilli.

Add the marinated chicken and stir fry until the chicken is tender on medium heat.

Add the vegetables: first carrots, after a minutes green beans and then the rest of the vegetables.

Don`t overcook the vegetables. When they are still crisp add corn flour and stir quickly for a minute.

Turn off heat, and take the wok off the stove You can serve this on a bed of plain white rice.

Prawn Chilli Fry

Prawns peeled: 1 cup
Onions: 3
Tomato paste: 1 can
Chilli powder: 1/2 or 1 tablespoon
Grated ginger: 1 teaspoon
Oil: 2 or 3 tablespoons
Apple cider vinegar: 1 1/2 tablespoons
Salt: 3/4 teaspoon

Pan fry prawns for two minutes or until they change color and set aside.

In a pan fry the onions cut thin elongated until light brown.

Add tomato paste, salt, grated ginger and chilli powder and fry for 5 minutes stirring constantly on medium heat.

Add the prawns and fry for another five minutes. Taste and add salt if needed.

Serve with rice, nan or brown pita bread.

Prawns with Potatoes

Prawns: 1/2 kg (1 lb, 1.64 oz)
Potatoes: 1 large
Onions: 2
Green Chillies: 1
Pepper: 1/4 teaspoon
Salt: 1/4 teaspoon
Tomato: 1
Coriander: 1 bunch
Olive oil: 2 tablespoons
Apple cider vinegar: 1 tablespoon

Peel and wash the prawns with salt and set aside.

Chop the onions, green chillies, coriander (1/2 bunch) and tomatoes.

Wash and cut the potato into small cubes and cook them in the microwave for 5 minutes with 1/2 cup of water or until they are done.

Fry the onions to golden brown in olive oil.

Add green chillies and tomatoes and fry for 5 minutes.

Add prawns, pepper, salt and vinegar and cook until the prawns are done. They change colour when they are done.

Add potatoes with the water and chopped coriander and bring it to a boil.

Taste and add salt if needed.

Fish Cutlets/Patties

Salmon or tuna: 1 can
Cabbage finely chopped: 1 cup
Potatoes: 2 (boiled and mashed)
Onions: 2 (finely chopped and fried into golden brown in 1tbs of olive oil)
Green chillies: 1 or 2 (finely chopped)
Coriander: 1/2 bunch finely chopped
Egg: 1 (beaten with a pinch of salt and set aside)
Vinegar: 1 tablespoon
Breadcrumbs or cream of wheat: 1 cup

Drain the water from the tuna or Salmon and set aside.

Fry onions to light brown.

Add chopped cabbage to the fried onions and cook with constantly stirring for 6/7 minutes.

Add chopped green chillies and coriander and fry for 2 minutes.

Add the mashed potatoes, tuna or salmon, pepper and salt.

Set aside until hot enough to handle.

Mix it with your hand. If you feel it is too watery to form cutlets add bread crumbs.

Form into round or oblong cutlets, dip each in the beaten egg and then cream of wheat (which should be spread on a plate) and fry on a non-stick pan with little oil until each side becomes brown.

Broiled Fish

Any fish fillets: 5
Chilli powder or pepper powder: 1/2 teaspoon
Salt: to taste
Vinegar or lemon juice: 1 tablespoon
Breadcrumbs or cream of wheat: 1/2 cup

Wash the fillets and pat dry with a paper towel and set aside.
Mix the ingredients.
Apply to each of the fillets.
Dip each one in the breadcrumbs or cream of wheat and place them in a greased pan.
Preheat oven 350 degrees.
Bake for 15 minutes or less depending on the thickness of the fish.

Prawns and Muscles in Wine Sauce

Prawns: 1/2 cup
Muscles: 1/2 cup
White wine: 1/2 cup
Butter: 1/2 tablespoon
Lemon: juice of 1/2 lemon
Pepper and salt to taste
Small onion: 1/2 (chopped very fine)

Wash, peel and dry the prawns and muscles and set them aside.
Fry the onion in the butter until light brown.
Add lemon, wine, salt and pepper and give it a boil. Add the prawns and muscles and boil until the liquid becomes about 1/4 cup.
Serve with multigrain bread and salad.

Prawn Vegetable Stir-fry

Whole wheat or rice pasta: 1 cup cooked
Prawns: 350 gm (12.36 oz)
Green pepper: 1
Red pepper: 1
Green onions: 2
Carrot: 1
Mushrooms: 4
Green Chilli: 1 finely chopped
Garlic: 1/4 teaspoon finely chopped
Vinegar: 1 tablespoon
Salt: 1/8 teaspoon
Olive oil: 3 tablespoons
Ginger grated: 1 teaspoon
Soy sauce: 2 tablespoons

Marinate peeled and cleaned prawns with chilli, ginger, garlic, vinegar, soy sauce and salt and set aside for 15 minutes.

Wash and cut vegetables into thin strips (about 1/2 inch).

Heat the oil and stir fry the prawn mixture, when prawns change colour, add carrots. After a minute or two, add the rest of the cut vegetables and stir-fry for another 5 or 6 minutes on high heat. Don't overcook veggies.

Add the cooked pasta or rice and mix well.

A wholesome meal is ready to eat.

Pork Chops

Pork chops: 6
Egg: 1
Ginger garlic paste 1/2 teaspoon
Bread crumbs
Chilly powder a pinch
Garam Masala: 1/2 teaspoon (get in an Indian store)
Salt: 1/4 teaspoon
Olive oil as needed

Marinate the pork chops with salt, chilly powder and ginger/garlic paste and garam masala for 1/2 an hour.

Dip each chop in the beaten egg and then roll in the bread crumbs and fry on a non-stick pan with some oil on medium heat.

Turn when the bottom side is brown and continue to fry until both sides are golden brown.

Spicy Pork

Boneless pork: 1/2 kg (1 lb, 1.64 oz)
Garlic: 1/2 cup chopped
Ginger: 1/2 cup chopped finely
Green chillies: 4 chopped finely
Paprika: 1 teaspoon
Salt: 1/2 teaspoon
Tomato paste: 1 can
Apple cider vinegar: 3 tablespoons

Wash and boil the pork in 3 cups of water for 10 minutes:(medium heat).

Take out the meat and cut it into small pieces (1" cubes).

Strain the water and set aside.

Rinse the pot and then add the strained water, cut pork and all the other ingredients except tomato paste and cook for half an hour on medium flame.

Add the tomato paste, mix thoroughly and cook for another 10 minutes.

Taste and add more salt or vinegar according to your taste.

You can eat it with rice or crusty brown bread

Beef-Chicken/Veal/ Chilly Fry

Stew beef/veal/chicken breast: 1 kg (2 lb, 3.274 oz)
Onions: 3
Tomato paste: 1 can
Chilli powder: 1/2 or 1 tablespoon
Grated ginger: 1 teaspoon
Oil: 2 or 3 tablespoons
Apple cider vinegar: 1 1/2 tablespoons
Salt 3/4 teaspoon
Water: 1 cup

Cut the meat or chicken into thin strips of about 2" long mix with apple cider vinegar and set aside.

In a pan fry the onions cut thin elongated until light brown.

Add tomato paste, salt, grated ginger and chilli powder and fry for 5 minutes stirring constantly on medium heat.

Add the meat or chicken and cook with water until it is tender on minimum heat.

Taste and add more salt if needed. Serve with rice, vegetables, nan or brown pita bread.

Keema or Ground Beef/Veal with Vegetables

Ground Beef/Veal: 500 gm (17.637 oz)
Onion: 1
Garlic/ginger paste: 1 tablespoon
Paprika: 1 tablespoon
Salt: 1/2 teaspoon
Coriander: 1/2 cup finely chopped
Carrot: 1 grated
Peas: 1/2 cup
Lemon juice: 2 lemons (juicy)
Tomato paste: 1 can
Apple cider vinegar: 1/2 tablespoon

Wear gloves and mix all ingredients with the ground beef with an exception of tomato paste and chopped coriander.

Cook for 35 minutes stirring regularly.

Add tomato paste and cook for 5 more minutes.

Garnish with chopped coriander.

Serve with rice, Chapatti, nan or crusty bread.

Ground Beef/Chicken/veal Patties

Ground beef/veal/chicken: 1 kg (2 lb, 3.274 oz)
Onions: 2 finely chopped
Green chillies: 2 long finely chopped or 1/2 teaspoon red pepper flakes
Garlic cloves: 4 finely chopped
Ginger: 1" skinned and finely chopped
Egg: 1 beaten
Breadcrumbs: 1/4 cup or more
Coriander: 1/2 cup finely chopped
Potato: 2 boiled and mashed
Oil: 2 tablespoons
Apple cider vinegar: 1 tablespoon
Salt to taste

Fry onions in 2 tablespoons of oil until light brown in a medium pot.

Add ground meat and continue to fry for at least another 10 minutes.

Add the chilli, garlic ginger and coriander and fry for 5 minutes.

Switch off the stove and let it cool.

Add some breadcrumbs

Once warm enough to handle, mix the mashed potatoes and mix with your hand.

Make patties according to the size you want.

Dip each patty in egg and then breadcrumbs and pan fry in a non-stick pan with minimum oil until both sides are nice and brown.

Serve with some vegetables, salad and good bread.

9

Snacks

Humus and Pita or Crackers

Chick peas (raw) washed and soaked overnight: 1 cup
Olive oil: 1 1/2 tablespoons
Tahini: 1/4 cup
Lemon juice freshly squeezed: 1/4 cup
Finely chopped garlic
Cumin: 1/2 teaspoon ground
Chilli, red (optional): 1
Salt to taste

Wash the soaked chickpeas and boil them with 2 cups of water on low heat until they are done. Note that the water has to be evaporated except for about 3 spoons.

You can use a can of chickpeas if this is too much work. Drain and wash the chick peas if they are canned. Add three spoons of fresh water.

Put the chickpeas with all the above ingredients in a blender and grind them slowly mixing often until it turns into a fine paste. You may add a bit of olive oil or water if needed.

Transfer to a bowl, garnish with paprika and wee bit of olive oil. Once this 'humus dip' is ready, you can use it with multi grain pita, crackers or vegetables as snack.

Grilled Sandwiches

Multigrain bread: 8 slices
Tomato: 1
Garlic clove: 1
Oregano: 1/2 teaspoon, dry

Green chilli (optional): 1
Swiss or any cheese: 4 slices
Olive oil: just enough to apply on both the sides of the griller
Sandwich griller for four sandwiches

Place the four slices on the sandwich griller.

Place the slices of cheese on them.

Mix the rest of the ingredients and spread them evenly on the four slices above.

Place the other four slices on the top of the spread.

Close the sandwich griller and place on medium heat on the stove for 5 to 7 minutes and then turn the griller and leave for another 5 minutes, so that the other side is done too.

Turn off the stove and remove the sandwiches.

Wait for 5 minutes and then cut each into four pieces.

You will have 16 mini sandwiches.

Dhokla: An Indian Dish

Semolina: 2 tablespoons
Yogurt: 1/4 cup
Chickpea flour: 1 cup
Lemon juice: 3 teaspoons
Grated ginger: 1/2 teaspoon
Chilli powder (optional): 1/2 teaspoon
Water: 1 cup
Eno Fruit Salt: 1 teaspoon
Salt to taste
Oil to grease the pan
Fresh grated coconut and chopped coriander leaves for garnish

Get the steamer ready on the stove with water boiling.

Place a pan or bowl which is at least 2" deep, that can fit into the steamer.

Mix all the ingredients except the Eno, coriander and coconut in a bowl.

Make sure the batter is smooth without any granules.

Once the batter is ready, add the Eno Fruit salt and briskly mix it with an egg beater for a minute.

Pour the batter into the pan in the steamer.

See that the batter is not more than 1/2 high, as it will rise when steamed.

Cover the steamer and steam for 10-12 minutes on medium heat.

Switch off the stove and let stand for a few minutes.

Cut the Dhokla into square pieces and garnish with fresh coconut and coriander. You should eat it with Chutney. That chutney can be also used to make sandwiches.

Chutney

Coconut, frozen or fresh: 1 cup
Coriander leaves: 1/2 cup
Green chillies (optional, you may put 1 or 2 according to your preference)
Garlic clove: 1
Cumin seed: 1/2 teaspoon
Lemon juice: (1/2 teaspoon) or small ball of tamarind
Salt to taste
Water: 1/8 cup

Grind all the ingredients in a blender or a bullet until it is a smooth mixture. Add salt or lemon according to taste.

Round Pumpernickel Bread and Dip

> Spinach: 1 bunch
> Light sour cream: 1 small container
> Garlic pod very finely minced: 1
> Green chilli finely minced (optional): 1 small
> Salt to taste

Carve the pumpernickel bread to make a round hole in the centre.

Leave only a thin layer of bread.

The carved bread should be cut into bite size pieces and arranged around the hallow shell and set aside.

Wash and cut the spinach leaves into tiny pieces and boil with a little bit of salt for only 5 minutes.

There should be no standing water in the spinach.

Mix it with sour cream and other ingredients.

Taste the salt and add if you need more.

Pour the mixture in the shell.

Your snack is ready to eat.

The same dip can be used to dip raw vegetables and crackers.

> "It's up to you today to start making healthy choices. Not choices that are just healthy for your body, but healthy for your mind."
>
> —Steve Maraboli, *Unapologetically You: Reflections on Life and the Human Experience*

Conclusion: Money

*M*oney plays an important part in our lives and most of us are not born with a lot of it. Hence, it is crucial that we plan our future with what is thrown at us. Being an inherently frugal Indian, I started saving as soon as I came to Canada and started working. When I was making only $5/hr, I still saved $50.00 a month which would be automatically withdrawn from my checking account on the first of every month. This way I had to live with what was left. The amount increased as I started earning more.

> "The habit of saving is itself an education; it fosters every virtue, teaches self-denial, cultivates the sense of order, trains to forethought, and so broadens the mind."
>
> —T.T. Munger

As my mother always said, "cut your coat according to your cloth," I learnt to live within my means and buy something only when I had enough money in the bank for it. I never bought things on credit unless it was absolutely necessary.

> "Financial peace isn't the acquisition of stuff, it's learning to live on less than you make, so you can give money back and have money to invest. You can't win until you do this."
>
> —Dave Ramsey

Having Economics and History as my major in university, I knew the difference between needs and wants and unlike the present generation of kids and adults who want 'instant gratification' of their wants, I learnt to put my limited means to satisfy the most important needs, first. In economics a need is defined as something you "have to have" and a want is something you "like to have." The wants in my life had to wait, as I decided to spend my limited resources on the needs of my family. A lot of sacrifice and determination went into this. This discipline helped me build my assets and have a reasonably comfortable retirement years. Financial independence reduces stress and contributes to a healthier life.

Death is an inevitable part of our existence and there is no escape from it no matter what we do. However, we can make this mortal life as happy and healthy as we can by what we feed our body, heart and mind and living our life fully and helping others along the way. Once we accept the fact that we are mortal and not push this thought away, we will be ready when the time comes. This will not stop us from living, but rather motivate and encourage us to live fully as we will be reminded that life is short.

The Dalai Lama has said that death is a part of all our lives. Whether we like it or not, it is bound to happen. Instead of avoiding thinking about it, it is better to understand its meaning. We all have the same body, the same human flesh, and therefore we will all die. There is a big difference, of course, between natural death and accidental death, but basically death will come sooner or later.

> "The fear of death follows from the fear of life. A man who lives fully is prepared to die at any time."
>
> —Mark Twain

Therefore let us live to the fullest and enjoy life, as long as our enjoyment is not at the expense of others' happiness. Hurt caused to innocent people will have its repercussions on our lives. It will rob us of our peace of mind and true happiness. Karma always has its reward or punishment.

> "You've gotta dance like there's nobody watching,
> Love like you'll never be hurt,
> Sing like there's nobody listening,
> And live like it's heaven on earth."
>
> —William W. Purkey